Lunches
with Ed

A Dementia
Journey *of* Love

Lunches *with* Ed

JUDY COLLIER

Lunches with Ed: A Dementia Journey of Love

Copyright © 2026 by Judy Collier. All Rights Reserved.

For information about this title contact the publisher:

Judy Collier
Collier.Judy23@gmail.com

ISBNs:
979-8-9995883-0-2 (softcover)
979-8-9995883-1-9 (eBook)

Printed in the United States of America

Cover and Interior design: 1106 Design

This book is dedicated to the many unsung family members
and friends who are caring for a loved one.

It is also lovingly dedicated to the memory
of my beloved husband, Ed.

Contents

Foreword

The events described within these pages are a true and accurate account. However, in an effort to preserve the anonymity of those mentioned herein, the names of characters and in some instances, places, have been changed.

Introduction

My husband Ed was diagnosed with dementia just about 15 years into our marriage. It was not the first marriage for either of us, but it was the union that was meant to be. At long last we had found each other. The trials and tribulations we had been through in our lives made us perfect for each other. We actually met at church, and the first time I noticed him I thought he was a very handsome man. Little did I know that he had already noticed me. I was not interested in meeting anyone, as I was divorced and decided that I would never ever get married again. I did not want to dive into that pool again. Well, as the saying goes . . . never say never.

When Ed first became incapacitated I tended to him at home until it became unsafe to do so, and I had to make the very difficult decision to place him in a skilled nursing home. The following is my accounting through journal entries I started making which was cathartic for me. There was laughter and tears. It is my hope that this chronicle will help others who may be entering this journey.

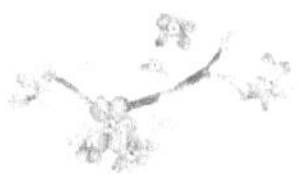

The Journey

I had been married for 15 years to Ed, the love of my life, when he was diagnosed with dementia. I knew from that point on, our day-to-day life would slowly change. I knew this as I was an onlooker when my father suffered from Alzheimer dementia and witnessed the changes my mother and sister went through as they cared for him. It seems there were many hospital trips for Ed almost immediately for physical ailments such as diverticulitis, UTIs, sepsis, c-diff and vertigo. These were hospital admittances that did not seem to be related to dementia. I started noticing things that my "handyman" around the house husband could no longer do. He did things like leaving the bathroom water running in the sink which led to flooding from the top floor down to the basement, or burning a pot while boiling eggs because the water had boiled away. He started getting lost while driving familiar routes. Once it took him two hours to get home from his brother Carlton's house which was a 20-minute drive, tops. Things like losing his phone, losing keys, leaving his wallet on an ATM, getting lost when driving home from Valley Forge casino and ending up in Lancaster County 50 miles away. The real clincher for me was when he could not fix the bathroom sink and I had to actually finish the job after he dismantled the pipes. Ed was known as the family "plumber." He could conquer any plumbing job, large or small. He was the "plumber" and his brother Carlton was the "carpenter." Between the two of them, the family never had to call a repairman to fix things around the house.

One night when driving home he had an accident with a SEPTA trolley. SEPTA, or the Southeastern Pennsylvania Transportation Authority, was the mass transit system in the area. He was shaken up and the car was damaged. Thank goodness he was not seriously hurt, although he spent several weeks in physical therapy for stiffness and aches. He blamed everything on SEPTA and wanted to sue for millions. He was obsessed with suing SEPTA not only because of the accident, but also because he had worked for them for years as a bus and high-speed trolley driver and was duped out of his fair pension. It seemed as though he was told he was not fully vested but later found out from fellow co-workers, who had the same amount of time as he had, they had gotten a huge check or monthly payments in their retirement. Ed had only gotten checks for several months and then they stopped. When I met Ed he had already retired from SEPTA and was working for tour bus companies. I never fully understood what the story was, but I believe it also had something to do with the union and maybe the union had fought for the co-workers. He was bitter, to say the least. Later after many phone calls to the insurance company, consultations with lawyers, viewing traffic video, it was evident that he had, in fact, been the culprit that caused the accident as he was driving in a restricted trolley lane.

It was after the accident with the SEPTA trolley that his doctor recommended he take an occupational driving course to ensure he was still driving safely. I had already picked up on several things Ed had started doing while he was driving that made me nervous as a passenger. If I said anything about his driving, he would shush me as he was a "professional" driver and it would lead to an argument, so I learned not to say anything. Ed and I almost never argued, so this was a real concern for me. Later on, I refused to ride in the car with him. It was too stressful for me, especially since I could not yell "look out" if needed! After the visit with the occupational driving therapist and subsequent driving test in live traffic, it was suggested that Ed give up his license. The therapist stated it was much better to do it voluntarily. Ed reluctantly gave it up and got a state identification card instead. This was somewhat a relief for me and I assured him that I would drive him anywhere he wanted to go. It was okay for a while. Then Ed became obsessed with getting his license back. I realized that being a bus driver was part of his identity, and the fact that he could no longer drive really worked on his psyche. What I didn't see coming was the fact that it also made me really depressed. It was a big adjustment for both of us. I was not as adventurous as Ed was when it came to driving places, whether near or far, and so we did not go as many places as we used to. He blamed the doctor that ordered the driving test for taking his license and kept saying that the doctor had his license in his desk drawer. He was mad at that doctor and refused to go see him again. I had to find another doctor which I hesitated to do because he was a good doctor and did not just rush us in and out whenever we went. Everything worked out, though, because I eventually found another general doctor as well as a neurologist that turned out to be heaven-sent for us. The neurologist was an older, caring man and knew exactly how to examine/treat Ed. He would ask Ed several questions while we both were in the room, then take Ed to another examining room and come back and ask me privately what was really going on. In his experience, he knew that patients often were less than honest when telling the doctor how good they are doing. (Ed would always tell doctors he was doing great.) He would also show genuine concern for me and how I was coping, explaining that I would probably need outside help as time went on.

Aside from Ed insisting he was going to get his license back, he also thought his car was parked somewhere several blocks away. The car he had to find was not one of the cars we had, but was a car he had years ago. A car he had before I even knew him. He insisted we go walking around the neighborhood to look for his car. So off we went walking. Ed had lived not too far away from where I lived when I met him. When we married, he sold his house and moved in the house I lived in, as it was smaller and more suitable for us as a couple. So we actually walked from our house back to his old house looking for a non-existent car. It was a nice walk on a pleasant weather-wise day, however, and somehow he was satisfied when we returned home and never brought the subject up again. The next obsession he had was wanting to go to the police station to report on a crime one of his buddies supposedly committed when they were teenagers. I don't know what it was but it was something that must have bothered him. So once again we leave the house, hop in the car, me driving, of course, under the guise of going to the local police station to report on a crime maybe committed 55–60 years ago. I drove around long enough to distract him and soon we were able to come back home.

It was not long after these incidents that all he wanted to do was stay in bed all day. He would sleep most of the day and didn't want to come down to eat. He would say he wasn't hungry, but if I took a plate up to him he would eat it. Sometimes I would have to feed him because it seemed he was too tired to feed himself. Our life became a series of doctor's appointments, labwork and visits to the hospital. I think I called the ambulance at least twice, once when he fell when he thought he could fly and jumped off the bed. Ed was on a blood thinner due to his AFib and the doctor had told us that if he ever falls he needed to go to the ER to make sure there was no internal bleeding. The other time I called was when he had a high fever and was nearly lethargic which was due to an undiagnosed UTI which turned into sepsis.

Once home from the hospital admission, health care teams would visit—PT, OT, nurses, social worker and a doctor. The social worker suggested senior day care which Ed eventually agreed to attend. Of course I had to tell him he was "going to work." When we first arrived at the center, I told the intake administrator that Ed thought he was going to work. She said that's okay because most of the attendees thought they were going to work as well, and that this was their job. He was anxious to go, even on days when he did not sleep very much at night. The senior day care was excellent for him. He engaged with the others there. There were games, trivia questions, conversations and a hot lunch provided every day. They even had a therapy dog "Penny," a copper-colored golden retriever that came once a week on Wednesdays. Ed loved animals and would enjoy petting and giving Penny treats. I was able to sit in and observe the daily routines whenever I wanted. When he came home from his "job" he would tell me all about what the fellas talked about at lunch. He said they all sat at the same table telling stories and jokes. He said there was one woman who always wanted to sit with the men and she was obsessed with her pocketbook. She was worried that someone was trying to take it. It tickled me that he knew and remembered the particulars of the day. The center worked out well for us. By the time he got home, we had a few hours before dinnertime and then bed. The center was a great solution. The respite I got while Ed was there afforded me time to go grocery shopping, go to the salon and even to get an occasional massage where I would dream I was on a tropical beach. This time was short-lived. The pandemic hit. It was March 2020 and everything was shut down.

It was surprising to me how fast Ed declined once the regimen of the center was gone. The staff attempted to keep up a home routine by sending packets to us . . . arts and crafts, puzzles and even supplying a YouTube link for exercises on video with the staff members Ed was accustomed to. We followed along for a while, but soon Ed was not interested and did not pay attention. Soon the periods of wanting to stay in bed all day and not wanting to eat, roaming around in the middle of the night began. This period was particularly challenging because of the isolation and fear caused by the pandemic. The unknown virus which was named corona virus 19 or Covid-19 created such turmoil, nobody knew what to do, and people were afraid to be around others as it was suggested by the government that people not socialize outside of their household members. The days and nights grew long. I tried doing puzzles with Ed at our dining room table. He would attempt to find the pieces but more times than not he would simply try to force a puzzle piece into a space to make it fit. Many pieces were getting bent and mangled. We soon stopped doing puzzles together.

Ed wanted to stay in bed all day as previously mentioned. He didn't want to bathe, get dressed or shave. He slept a lot during the day and through the night. At some point, he started waking up in the middle of the night and would roam around the house looking for his kids. His kids were grown and they had kids of their own. In his mind they were still young children, around 10 or 11 years old. Plus, he was obsessed that one of his daughters was in trouble and needed his help. He started disassembling ceiling light fixtures, actually standing on a wobbly bed, reaching up to the light, removing the cover, bulbs and pulled the wires out. He thought his kids were up there. Once he tore up the guest room: Furniture was overturned and he had started to rip off the underside felt covering of the box spring looking for his son. I woke up just in the nick of time to prevent total destruction. Another evening he went down into the basement, found a ladder and removed the ceiling tile and climbed up into the opening so that he was looking at the floor of the room above. He thought his son was trapped between the floors. Trapped between the living room and the basement. I had to coax him down which led to his anger and defiance. I then had to hide the ladder so he could not do that again. Once he got an idea in his mind, he was hell-bent on carrying through on whatever it was. He walked around looking for that ladder for quite a while. I had hidden it behind the dining room table until I could take it out to the backyard the next morning. Did I mention this was in the middle of the night? We both were in our pajamas.

This was Ed's wandering period. It became really dangerous when he started going outside the house in the middle of the night. I had motion detector lights, door locks, cameras and apps to alert me when he got out of the bed at night. I had to sleep with one eye open. My phone would alert me whenever the front door opened. One night my phone went off and when I looked at it, I saw Ed coming back into the house. In my exhausted state, I had not heard the phone ding when he went out. I had no idea how long he had been outside the house. It was 3:00 a.m.

On another occasion he ran outside after pushing me away from blocking the door. He ran around the house to the backyard to the border of our yard and was talking to a bush like it was a person. He would not come back into the house. I was afraid he would wake up our neighbors. This too was a middle of the night episode. I had to call the police for assistance. This was done with much reluctance, considering how some police respond. I was afraid that all the police would see was a man, a prowler, wandering around suspiciously in the middle of the night. My social worker friend who works with dementia cases told me if I ever had to call the police, to repeat over and over he has dementia, he has dementia. When the cop arrived, to my surprise, he was very nice and said he understood what I was going through because he was going through the same thing with his mother-in-law. He also said that I'm going to have to do something. This was the second time I had to call them. He added before he left that I should not hesitate to call them back if necessary and that he was on duty all night. This was 3:00 a.m. again.

The first time I called the cops was when he was erratically destroying things inside the house and would not stop. There were times when I was afraid.

One night I decided to sleep on the couch because I figured Ed could not get out the front door without me hearing him. Well, when I woke up, Ed was coming back into the house. This was during the day, during the Covid-19 pandemic. I had no idea if he had come in contact with another person or not. I was doing my best to keep us both safe so as not to be exposed, and here he was, walking outside to who knows where. It was after these many instances and unsafe behavior that I decided I indeed needed to do something. I started looking for a facility.

Ed was admitted to a long-term care facility I'll refer to as SH in June 2020 during the pandemic. The pandemic started in March and was thought to be only a two-week shutdown. It ended up lasting two years, and even when things started reopening, it was advised to wear N-95 facial masks. This was a scary time in our history. The entire first year of Ed's stay was during the pandemic. It was a hard decision for me to make, but I knew I could not care for him at home and did not trust a slew of aides coming and going in the house. I felt he would be safer in a closed, controlled environment. One of the aides I had used while Ed was home informed me that her agency had told them to not wear masks when they went to various houses. That did not sit well with me. I also knew of a fellow church member that informed me his mother-in-law got Covid from her aide that came to the house while knowing she was sick. So I had to put my trust that the good Lord would watch over and protect my husband.

Inside visitation was not allowed during this period. I had to schedule window visits to see Ed. An aide would bring him downstairs to the first floor lounge area which was surrounded by huge floor-to-ceiling windows. There was a patio area around the back where I would talk to Ed on a phone while looking at him through the window. I also made a card with a red heart that said I Love You that I would hold up to the window for him to see. We would talk about anything, everything and nothing. It was just good to see him. Once he was there and was acclimated to things, sometimes he would cut the visit short, saying he wanted to get back to the daily activity, whatever that was. Once he even just said, "Well nice seeing you, I'll talk to you later." Oh no, he didn't just dismiss me! It was good in a way that he was adjusting, but still, I couldn't believe he just dismissed me. When my father was diagnosed with dementia, I remember the doctor telling my mother that sometimes families wait too long to place their loved one in a facility and the patient never adjusts, and it's better to place them a little too early than a little too late. I sometimes think I could have kept Ed home a little longer, and had it not been for the pandemic I may have; but I had started to hear stories of how it was difficult finding in-home help, not to mention the non-mask wearing of the aides, as mentioned previously. I sure didn't want to bring Covid into my house.

So during that first year, I faithfully scheduled window visits with Ed and also had phone care conferences with the team of professionals that tended to him. This included the social worker, nurse, physical therapist, occupational therapist and dietician. They kept me informed of his progress, daily routine and habits, whether he was eating, participating in the activities and socializing with others. They said he loved to sing and even sent me a video of him singing along in one of the group activities. In addition to the window visits, soon FaceTime phone calls and Zoom calls were available. That added extra visits with Ed. The calls were limited to 30 minutes, but sometimes the aide would leave the phone or tablet with Ed for longer periods and we just enjoyed that time. Once Ed had the phone while he was in the activity room and he spun the phone around so that I could see the room full of residents as they listened and sang along to Motown songs. The activity assistant even introduced me to the group and played a song in my honor. She first played "My

Girl" by the Temptations, and then she said she had to play the answer to the song for Ed and played "My Guy" by Mary Wells. I came to know the assistant via these video calls first and later in person. She was such a wonderful, caring person. One of the male residents that was sitting next to Ed while we had a video call overheard our conversation and said he wish he had someone to call him like that. He heard Ed and me professing our love for each other. He told Ed he was lucky. I found out later that Ed would brag to the guys that he had a beautiful wife. The video calls also afforded me a chance to see Ed's room. I had to send personal effects in by the aides and had to entrust them to place photos and such to make his room seem more welcoming for him.

The Zoom calls became a great tool for us to visit. Many times, Ed would be in his room, and as he did not have a roommate then, we could have private conversations, laugh and sing as we pleased. I would also turn my camera around so that he could see the cat I had adopted. Ed and I always had a cat or two throughout our marriage. I had Higgins when we first got married. Then we had Chloe after Higgins passed. We ended up with two cats, Chloe and Jasmine, when my son decided he was moving from New York to Los Angeles and wanted me to take in his cat. Jasmine in effect became Ed's cat. She took to Ed and followed him around and many times would end up sleeping on his chest while he lounged in the living room chair. I think Jasmine was used to a male human parent and that is why she took to Ed so easily. So I referred to Chloe as my cat and Jasmine as Ed's cat. Both cats enjoyed long lives under our care. I adopted Sydney during the pandemic after Ed was placed, even though I had stated I would not get another cat. Sydney became my companion during the long, lonely days during the shutdown. Ed never saw Sydney in person, so I would show him over the video whenever he came into the room while I was talking to Ed. Ed would get a kick out of watching him, especially when Sydney looked directly right at the camera.

Ed and I got into a regular rhythm of window visits, FaceTime and Zoom calls. On his first birthday while there, I set up a Zoom meeting with all his children. Ed's birthday was right around the Christmas holiday so I had to make sure they would all be available, and I did not want to interfere with their holiday time with their individual families. It turned out to be a good meeting. They all got to see and talk to Ed and also to see each other. Even though all but one of them lived locally, they did not really stay in touch with each other. It was like a family reunion on Zoom. We shared stories and they talked to each other as much as they talked to Ed. Of course we ended up singing happy birthday to him, the traditional song and the Stevie Wonder version. Ed was somewhat attentive, sometimes closing his eyes and appearing to not be listening. I actually recorded that meeting and would listen to it sometimes. It was just about 30 minutes long. I actually recorded a few of our video calls and took still pictures of the screen. Some nights when I had trouble sleeping I would replay the audio of the calls. It was comforting to hear his voice and the laughter we would share doing those calls. I am so glad that I thought to make those recordings. They are still on my phone and I also made a backup copy of them on a thumb drive. These are memories I will always have.

On January 24, 2022, SH started allowing inside visitation. First the inside visits were confined to the first floor lounge area where the seating was arranged at safe distances from others. On warm days I could take Ed outside where I could find a nice private area so we could spend time together. These outside visits would continue even after the facility opened up. Later as the pandemic was getting under control and vaccines were available, daily visits were allowed in the café on the fourth floor. That was the floor that Ed was assigned to, the locked, dementia floor. The elevator freely took you up to this floor, but in order to leave the floor, you had to enter a code to operate it. This was so that the residents on the floor would not try to leave unless accompanied by staff or family. Occasionally, visits were allowed in his room, as long as he did not have a roommate, or later, if he had one, could not be in the room.

When Ed first arrived at the facility he was ambulatory, albeit a little off-balance. He had started using a walker to walk down the hallway the week of April 18, 2022. Later as he regressed to wheelchair use, he could roll himself down the hallway.

He liked Ana (a social worker) and liked to give her a kiss on the cheek. Ana was the first person I met at SH. She was a kind, caring person, and I would always look forward to seeing her daily too. Other staffers were:

Tony—male aide that Ed referred to as the little boy because he was maybe 5'4".

Amber—fourth floor unit coordinator.

Naomi and Ruth—social workers, Ruth also belonged to the church Ed and I went to at that time.

Rocky—van driver.

All the wonderful nurses on that floor—Yvonne, Tatiana, Charlotte and others.

Aides—Miss B, whom Ed developed a close relationship with. She was wonderful with him.

Miss Sonya, the activity assistant.

There were many other wonderful aides and staff that I grew to know during my daily visits.

You will notice that there are sometimes long gaps between my journal entries. Many days I did not write. Many days I was exhausted. This reflects the hectic world I involuntarily entered into. I did not think to start a journal of my visits until many months after Ed's admittance.

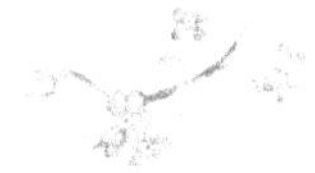

Journal Entries

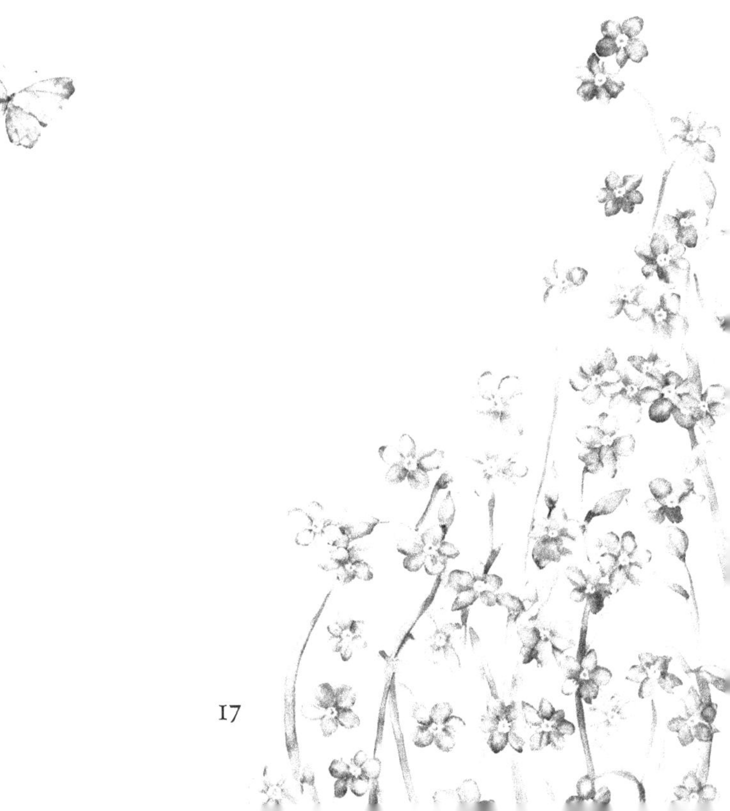

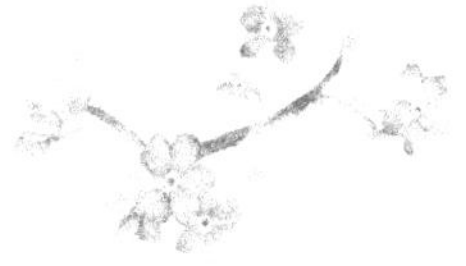

April 29, 2022

Ed rolled himself all the way down the hallway today in his wheelchair using his feet to assist. He was half asleep and ate half of his lunch today. Fish on Friday. He was not talkative at all. When I said I would help him eat when I finished my salad, he said "Uh oh, you shouldn't have told me that because now I'm gonna wait."

Today I found out he could no longer sign his name. Just scribbled. I was trying to get him to sign something that came in the mail. He could not. He seemed quiet and a little sad today . . . although happy at first. There are days when I visit him he tears up and tears run down his cheeks. This morning while I was home before I got dressed to visit him, I had a crying spell. It seems so hopeless at times. I put up a strong, happy facade, but just below the surface, there is sadness and fear. When Ed tears up, I think he knows, feels fear and trapped that he can't do or express himself. I know he knows I love him and he loves me and still tells me so. I make sure he knows and feels my love for him. Some days we just sit holding hands, usually with music playing on my iPhone-SiriusXM or Amazon Prime Music. Ed loves it when I rub lotion on his arms, legs and feet. He says hmmm as I am doing it and I know he enjoys it. He also likes the neck and back rubs I give him.

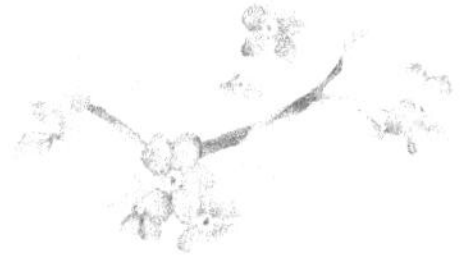

May 2, 2022

Today while having lunch with Ed, I mentioned that Mother's Day was coming up on Sunday and said I missed my mom. I asked him if he remembered her, and he said yeah with a big smile on his face. I reminded him he took mom to some of her doctor's appointments. He remembered that and then asked, "I wonder how she gets to her doctor appointments now?" I just said, "I'm sure she's all right."

I did not see any point in telling him Mom passed in 2011. No sense in risking him getting upset or sad. Ed was a little nonsensical today with some things he was telling me, but still we were able to enjoy each other's company. We laughed, held hands and sang along with some songs playing on my iPhone. Al Green was one of Ed's favorite singers and he would loudly sing "Let's Stay Together," "Love and Happiness," or "Tired of Being Alone," one of our favorites. I think we both liked that one because we had read somewhere that Al Green wrote that song in the wee hours of the morning in about 30 minutes when his girlfriend was not around.

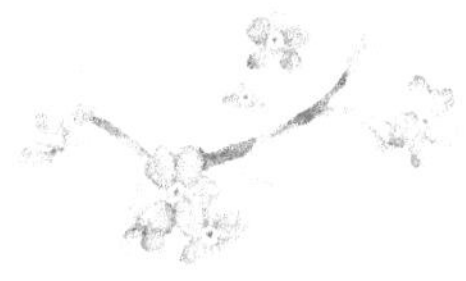

May 7, 2022 Saturday

The other day, I think it was Thursday, Ed had his eyes closed most of the time during my visit. I told him he didn't love me anymore because he never looks at me. He said, "I don't need to look at you because you are in my portfolio book and I know what you look like." Ha-ha—his eyes still closed!

A lot of days were like this. I learned how to carry on one-sided conversations. I would talk for long periods of time while he would just say um-hum. I became quite a storyteller. I don't know where those stories came from. I would just make up things to talk about. I found myself just doing anything to let him know I was there, to show him my love and care for him. Awhile back, Ed had asked me if we were still married. I assured him YES, we are in this together and I am not going anywhere. I think he was confused because he was no longer living in our house, and I also think someone at the facility may have put that thought in his head. He was pleased that I told him WE ARE STILL MARRIED.

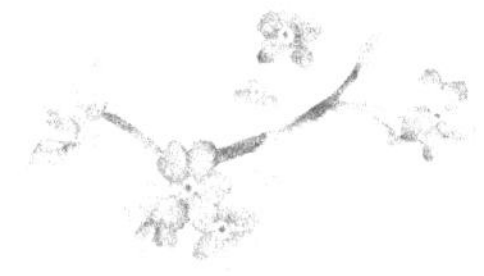

May 9, 2022 Monday

Today I had a wonderful visit with Ed. He was very talkative. He had just come from physical therapy. The therapist said he did wonderful today while Ed said he did terrible simultaneously. He told me he didn't see me for two days (and he was right). I had meetings on Saturday, and Sunday was Mother's Day so I decided not to add to the congestion that would be there that day. (Remember we were still following Covid-19 protocol). He looked so healthy and happy. His complexion was rosy and his skin so smooth. Although his conversation was coherent most of the time, it was intermingled with things that were not. He claimed that he had visitors earlier in the day of whom I knew were already dead. One was a lady that lived upstairs from his childhood home, Mrs. Lars. He would also say that he saw his brother Jake or sister Frankie. Jake was his older brother who had passed away 12 years prior. I had never met his sister Frankie because she had passed before I met Ed.

He would sometimes mistake one of the aides that worked there for a friend from his old neighborhood, a lady named Verna. I met Verna years ago when Ed took me to visit her. She still lived in the old neighborhood then. (She was known for her delicious homemade pound cakes. I can almost taste it now as I think about it). Ed ate at his own pace today starting with ice cream first. I just let him enjoy it any way he wanted today. He was a little confused as to where he was, one time asking me if I had been to other bases. I guess he thought we were on an army base. He also asked me if I had a key to the place. Despite everything, I really treasure these times with Ed. My love for him is so strong. We laughed, talked, hugged and held hands. I love this man more and more every day. What we have, most people never experience.

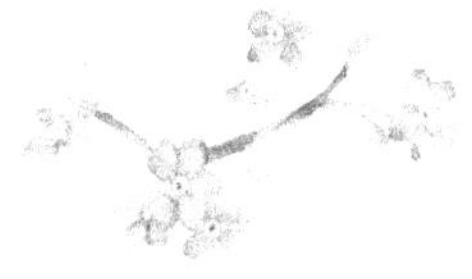

May 12, 2022 Thursday

Today was an off day for Ed. He was in his room in bed the entire time I was there. He was upset when I first arrived, saying there were two men there and they were going to be convicted. He thought he was going to be convicted too for something. I told him he was a good man and didn't do anything wrong to get convicted. He asked how did I know. I assured him everything was going to be all right. At one point he had tears welling up in his eyes. I comforted him as best I could and soon he was okay. Then I rubbed lotion on his arms, legs and feet. He always liked that. His eyes were closed most of the time I was there. I did get him to eat a good portion of his meal though: mac and cheese, BBQ chicken, broccoli, ice cream and pie. I was surprised he ate that much. He let me feed him, opening his mouth obediently for more. He went into a deep sleep after eating so I kissed him and quietly left the room.

After such a great day on Monday, he had been mostly sleepy the rest of the week. The nurse told me yesterday that he was agitated and didn't want to take his meds or get dressed. He was pushing and shooing the aides away. This was not like him. He was usually friendly and easygoing. Despite this terrible disease, he was kind and considerate. One of the female residents had a lifelike baby doll that she had left in the common area. Ed had found it and was walking around trying to find out who it belonged to. The nurse said he was carrying it the proper way, cradling it like a newborn baby. That was an example of his kindness.

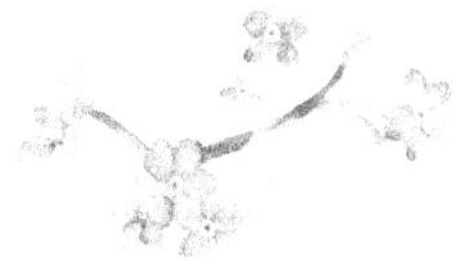

May 14, 2022 Saturday

Today I got a phone call from Ed's second daughter. She had just visited her dad as she does every other Saturday. She wants to take her mother to visit Ed. Her mother and Ed divorced over 40 years ago. I told her NO. I was thinking, why now??? I had become very protective of Ed. It was not that I had anything against the ex, I actually liked her. It was more of the daughter who wanted her mother to see her father and I'm sure she suggested it. Not to mention, she had told me her mother had dementia. I may have been wrong, but I thought it was not a wise thing to do. It wasn't just her, I did not want any unnecessary visits from people. First of all, if it wasn't someone who saw Ed on a regular basis, why visit him now when he was incapacitated? Secondly, there are people that just want to visit so that they can go back and "report" to others just how bad off someone is doing. Just being nosy. I hate to say there are a lot of so-called church folk who are guilty of the latter. I did not tell many people what facility Ed was in just for this very reason. I did not want people who were mere acquaintances of Ed to see him. That is the problem when someone is placed in a long-term care facility. Even though visitors have to sign in, almost anyone can go at any time, whether the resident wanted to see them or not. I'm sure he would not have wanted many people to see him in that state. I felt it was my job to protect Ed from needless intrusions.

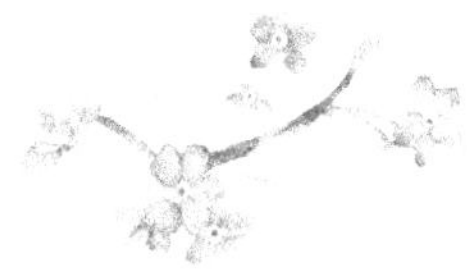

May 31, 2022 Tuesday

It was a good day with Ed. After eating lunch, we sat in the café and looked out the window at the scenery and cars passing by on the hill. We laughed, hugged and even sang a little with the songs playing on my iPhone. Precious moments.

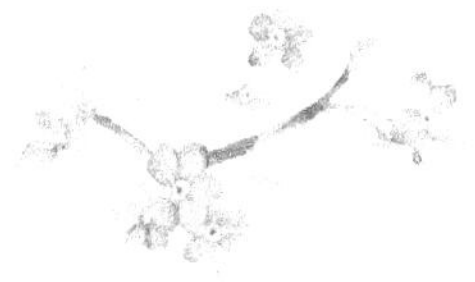

June 19, 2022 Sunday
Father's Day

I went to visit Ed today and took him a gift from his oldest daughter that she had dropped off to me on Thursday. Ed ate a little bit of his food. I took a picture of him holding the gift, which was a shirt, and texted it to his daughter. Shortly after that, he got sick and threw up all the food he had just eaten. His favorite aide, Miss B, came and got him, cleaned him up and then he got in bed. Evidently his system was backed up and everything came out (both ends). Irregularity is a common problem due to lack of activity. He felt better after that and just wanted to rest . . . understandable. I sat with him for a few hours. The TV was on and I found a gospel show to watch with him. After he went into a deep sleep, I quietly left the room.

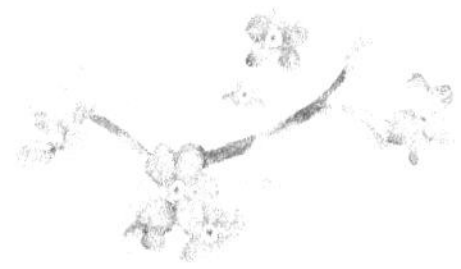

June 21, 2022 Tuesday

At lunch today, Ed did not eat a thing. He sat in the wheelchair with his eyes closed the whole time. He liked it when I gave him a couple of tight, long hugs.

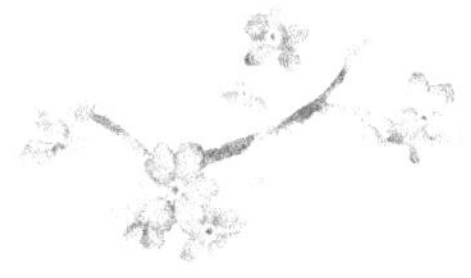

July 2, 2022

I went to visit Ed today. He looked really good. Every day at lunch when his food comes I say, "Let's say grace" and I usually ask if he wants to say it or if he wants me to say it. I usually say it. Well today when his food came, HE said, "Let's say grace" and proceeded to pray. I was so elated, I couldn't believe it! Thank you, Lord. Praise God.

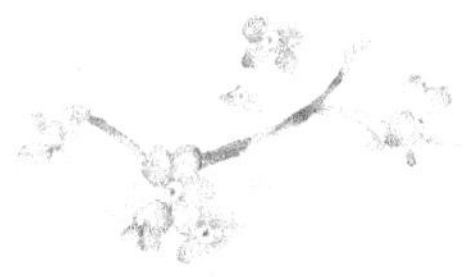

July 8, 2022

I took Ed some cut-up watermelon chunks which he really enjoyed. He spit a little white seed out and it landed on the table. I started telling him something and he said, "Oh, I thought you were going to say something about that" as he picked up the seed that landed on the left side of the tabletop. I looked at him and told him, "You knew that was wrong," and he started laughing.

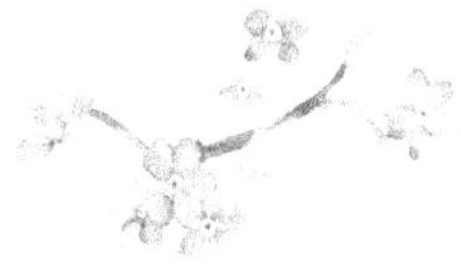

July 12, 2022 Tuesday

Today while Ed and I were in the café, in walks Deacon Clifton from our church, Zion Baptist. He is so energetic and positive. Ed was happy to see him and lit up with a big smile. Ed ate almost all of his food while Clifton was there and even offered him something to eat. Clifton was talking and telling us funny stories. He said his neighbor has chickens and he teases them by playing rooster sounds on his phone. He said the chickens pause and look around as if looking for the male.

He is so funny. Before leaving, he said a wonderful prayer, blessing Ed and me and then sang a song. After he left, Ed and I sat outside in the gazebo for about 45 minutes. What a wonderful visit it was today.

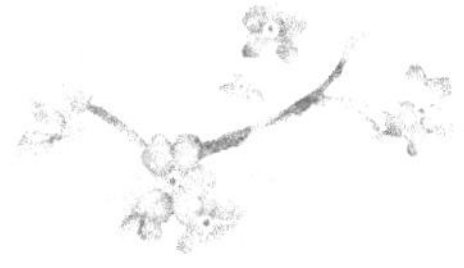

July 23, 2022

I went to visit Ed a couple of evenings this past week instead of at lunchtime.

He was already in bed with his dinner tray still there. We watched part of the movie *Cincinnati Kid* starring Steve McQueen before he drifted off to sleep. One other night he asked me to pray before I left. Praying and reciting Psalm 23 became my departing routine. It brought a peaceful calmness to both of us.

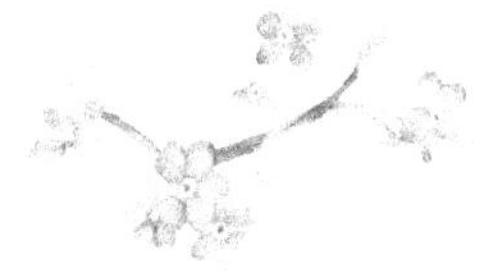

July 29, 2022 Friday

Today at lunch, Ed separated the grapes I brought him into groups of four. I don't know why but he was concentrating on getting it right. I brought him red grapes every day and sometimes apple slices or a banana. We then ate the grapes in groups of four, he starting on one end and me on the other end. He didn't want any of his lunch today, only one belVita biscuit and soda. We went outside after lunch and sat in the sun, listening to music. Ed and I spent many days outside when the weather permitted. It gave us much-needed privacy and a chance to get fresh air and sunshine.

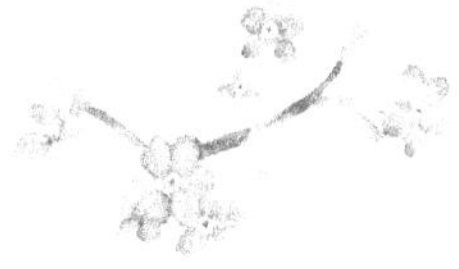

August 25, 2022

Today I was told that Ed's roommate tested positive for Covid and was taken to the hospital. I became worried for the two of us because the day before, the actual day the roommate went to the hospital, Ed and I ate in the café and Ed actually insisted that I taste his food and so I tasted it using his fork. Oh no, I'll never do that again. Ed was tested and he was negative.

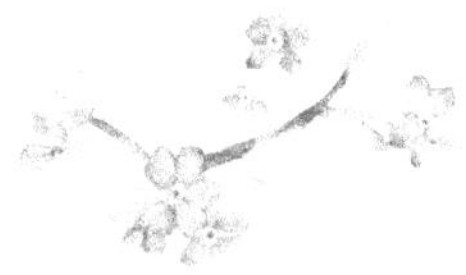

August 29, 2022

I went to visit Ed on Sunday. I stayed away a few days pending additional Covid tests. I also self-tested and was negative twice. Ed also tested negative twice.

Sunday he was rather tired and although he ate, he only ate if I fed him. He said he was feeling fine and nothing was hurting or bothering him. It is rather disappointing that he has a roommate now because that means I can no longer go into his room . . . Covid rules.

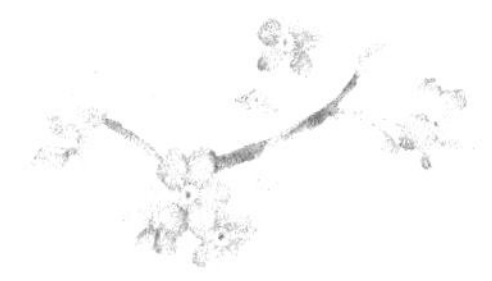

September 21, 2022

Today Ed told me to, "Quit talking and git to walking." Context—he was tired and didn't want to eat, he just wanted me to take him back to his room so he could sleep.

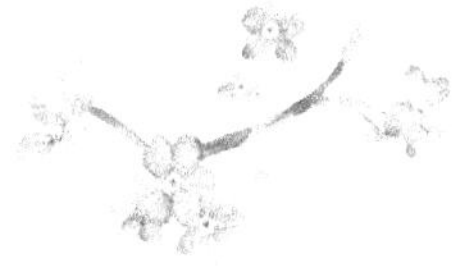

November 23, 2022

Today when I went to visit Ed for lunch, he navigated his wheel-chair all the way down the long hallway from his room to the café. He used his arms, hands and feet to direct the chair. He turned in to the café and was able to pull right up to the table. I made a video of him doing this. Once he got situated at the table, he looked at me and asked, "Where are you going to sit?" I told him, "Right beside you." We sat at the same table with a friend I had met while she visited her mother who was also a resident. We were usually there every day at the same time. The fact that Ed was able to work his wheelchair the way he did was evident that the physical therapy and occupational therapy he was getting was effective.

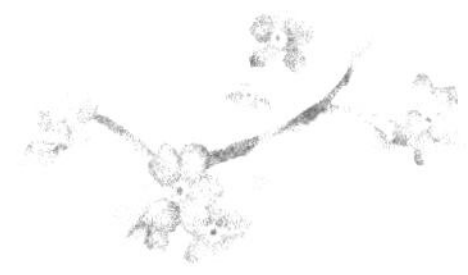

November 28, 2022

SH has been under new management, new owners effective October 1ˢᵗ. I started going over almost every day without fail. Initially I was worried because I wasn't sure if the care level would remain up to par. The facility went from being nonprofit to a for-profit facility. So far, things appear to be status quo. Most of the caregivers and all of the nurses caring for Ed are still the same and I know all of them. Ed is content, but his dementia is at a different stage now. He sleeps a lot and his appetite has decreased.

I was able to visit Ed in his room whenever his roommate wasn't there. As I was visiting, I said, "I don't know why (and before I could say "my shoulder was hurting") he said, "There's no sun up in the sky"—Lyrics to the song "Stormy Weather."

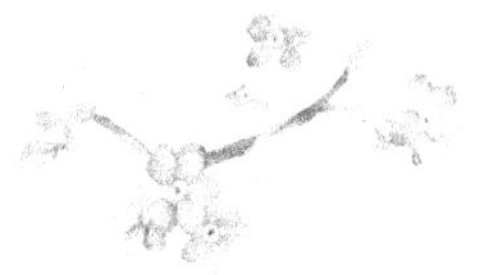

February 8, 2023

Lately Ed has been pretty stable. Today he was sleepy and didn't interact too much with me. This past Sunday (2/5/23) was a wonderful day with him. He was very alert. First we sat in his room listening and singing along to music. He was singing "Someone to Watch Over Me" and said, "I don't know how I know this song but I do." I told him I really liked that song and that my mother used to like it too. Then I got up from sitting on the side of the bed and went to the chair in his room to zip up my tote bag which I had left open there. Ed noticed what I did and asked why I did that. I just said I'd rather have it zipped up so people can't look in it (in case an aide came into the room). He said that was bothering him too. I was surprised he was even paying attention!

Later we went downstairs for the church service with Rev. Hucks. The facility had church services every Sunday and rotated different ministers each week. Ed was dozing a lot during the service but sang loudly "On Christ the solid rock I stand . . .

all other ground is sinking sand." He got very emotional, tears streaming down his face. At the end of the service, he wanted to talk to the minister. Rev. Hucks came to him and Ed told him he felt lost and confused. Rev. Hucks told him wonderful words of comfort and said he had nothing to fear because he was saved. "Trust God, we will all be with him if we believe," he said. He then said a really nice prayer for us. I believe Ed felt better after that. I think he was really expressing that he was fearful of death. The minister reassured him that those who are saved never really die because they go home to be with the Lord, and no one really knows when they will die but we all will.

As I was leaving SH, I ran into Herbert, a well-known minister of music in the area, who was sitting in his car with a female reverend. The words they spoke to me brought tears to my eyes. It was so spiritually led and heartfelt. What resonated even more was that the messages I heard that day starting with my daily prayer phone call, Sunday school, Alfred Street Baptist Church sermon by Pastor HJW and the sermon by Rev. Hucks all tied together. I joined the historic Alfred Street Baptist Church during the pandemic online, even though it was located in Alexandria, VA. It was a great source of comfort and support for me.

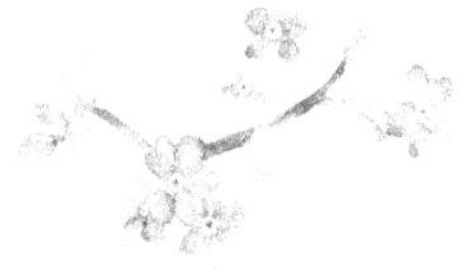

February 19, 2023

Today I took Ed down to the second floor for the church service. I enjoyed the services there too. It was the only service I was attending in person these days. Since the pandemic, I was watching church services online. The service today was led by a female minister who was very good. She always included lots of singing. Ed sang loudly, "I know it was the blood, I know it was the blood, I know it was the blood for me, one day when I was lost HE died on the cross, I know it was the blood for me."

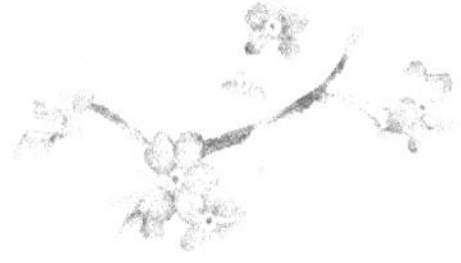

March 12, 2023

Today when I visited Ed we sat in the common area watching videos on the big-screen TV while waiting for the church service to start on the second floor. However, we never made it downstairs. The minister of music we knew from our community was there and started playing the piano on Ed's floor. He was a good friend of Ed's and Ed also knew his brother very well as they had worked together. As we started singing, others on the floor gathered around. People getting off the elevator to visit their loved ones stopped and joined in too. Ed would be singing loudly, "Pass Me Not" (Do Not Pass Me By), "Blessed Assurance" and "In the Garden."

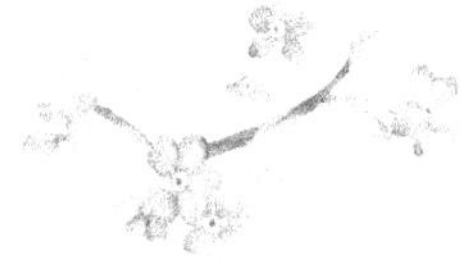

May 3, 2023

I had a care conference with Ed's team of caregivers at SH on Tuesday, April 25th. He was not eating and was continually losing weight. He is down to 154lbs. He stood at 5'11" and usually weighed around 185-190 lbs, and at one point was close to 200lbs. It was recommended that he start hospice. That word made me cry. He had been in and out of the hospital on numerous occasions by this point. I had witnessed the torture he went through in the ER and as an inpatient as they ran a gambit of tests, probed and poked. Droves of doctors and nurses constantly entering the room and asking the same questions over and over again. I had to be there because Ed could not answer the questions. The ER hospital staff was only concerned about treating the issue at hand and not considering the overall picture.

During my visit with Ed later back at SH, he was hallucinating and was fearful of people he saw in the corner of his room. He said they wanted to fight him. I walked over to the corner and talked out loud, very animated, to the imaginary people, telling them to leave Ed alone and to stop bothering him. I then told Ed that everything was okay, they will not bother you again. He was satisfied and calmed down. One of my new friends at the facility, the one who normally shared our lunch table along with her mother, was passing by Ed's room and saw me talking to the corner and wondered what I was doing. I told her that I had learned to enter into Ed's world and not try to convince him that no one was there. She said she would have never thought to do that. Her mother was in the room right next door to Ed's so she had similar scenarios to deal with.

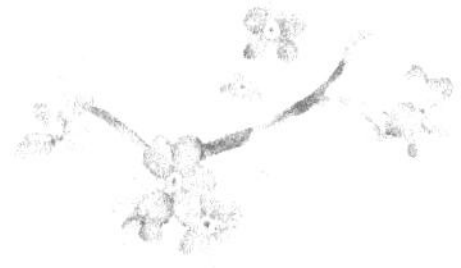

May 14, 2023

Ed was officially placed in hospice on Tuesday, May 9th. The hospice service provided another level of care. Right away a reclining wheel chair was delivered, an air mattress that automatically inflated and deflated periodically to prevent pressure points, and an aromatherapy lamp that softly misted the room . . . everything to keep him comfortable. One day I happened to arrive when the music therapist was there. She was playing the harp with its angelic sounds. He was sleeping lightly while she played "How Great Thou Art." I gently held his hand and rubbed his arm as she continued to play other hymns. It was such a peaceful setting. I needed to hear that harp. It brought comfort to me as well.

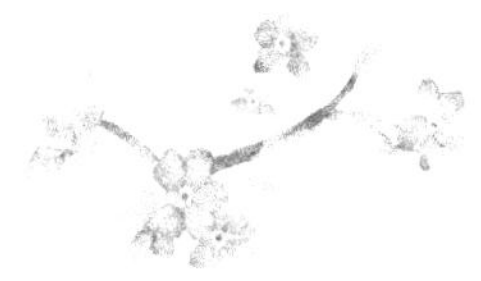

November 22, 2023

My beloved Ed passed away peacefully on June 4, 2023. I was with him when he took his last breath. I kissed him several times on his lips.

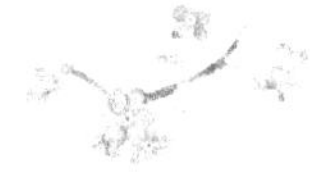

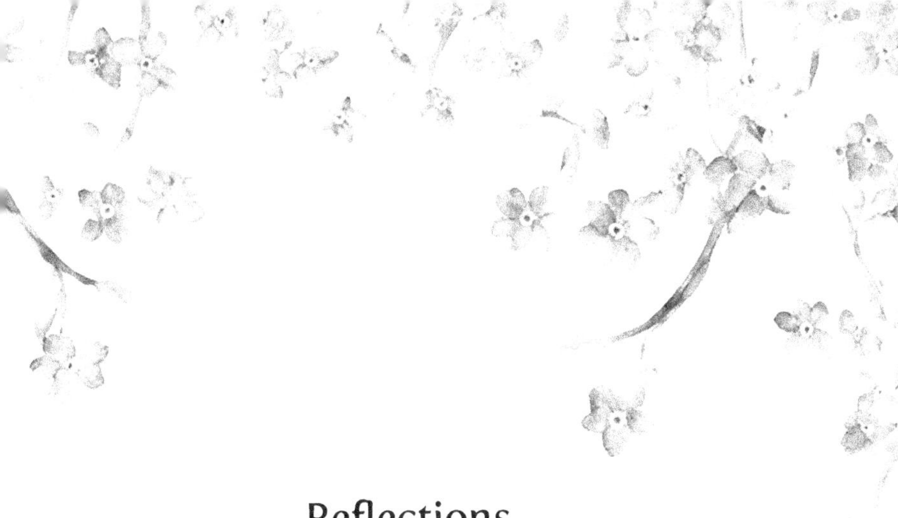

Reflections

May families have members that are diagnosed with dementia. This is a debilitating disease that affects all in its orbit. The disease is progressive and sometimes it moves fast (months) and sometimes moves very slow (years) until its terminal outcome. It takes the family or caregiver on a journey that can be as unique as the grooves of their fingerprints.

To prepare for my caregiving role I used many resources. I watched online videos of experts on the topic. A good source were videos by Teepa Snow, who offers a Positive Approach to Care found on YouTube. There are so many online resources nowadays. I read books such as *The 36-Hour Day* by Nancy L. Mace, MA, and Peter V. Rabins, MD, MPH; and *Coach Broyles' Playbook for Alzheimer's Caregivers* by J. Frank Broyles. I started attending support groups before Ed's symptoms appeared. After Ed was placed in long-term care, I found another support group for caregivers with loved ones in a facility. You are still a caregiver and also become an advocate once your loved one is placed. The actual hands-on day-to-day duties may change, but you are still totally involved. I chose to still do Ed's laundry. I felt that helped me maintain a closeness to him and also gave me an idea of his decline based on how soiled his clothes were. I also took him foods he liked on a regular basis. I accompanied him to specialist doctor appointments and did not rely on the staff to take him.

It was a learning process as I went along. What worked for me may not work for you. Flexibility is key. As mentioned in my journal entries, I had to adapt and enter into Ed's world. You cannot convince them they do not see or hear what they think they see or hear. I had to find ways to placate Ed and sometimes had to resort to a little "white lie." There was a period of time when Ed wanted to call 9-1-1 repeatedly. I had my brother-in-law and his wife call the house and pretend they were the police and would address his "urgent matter." That appeared to work. Later when Ed asked me if that was really the police, I reassured him that it was.

A big key is to learn the beauty of distraction. Whenever he was focused on doing something harmful, destructive or just inconvenient, I would distract him with something else. Sometimes it worked, sometimes it didn't. That's when being flexible comes in to play. That's when learning as you go along comes in to play.

Flexibility also includes the ability to admit and recognize when you need help. You cannot do it alone. I realized I needed help when it literally became unsafe for Ed to remain in the house. There were times I feared for my safety as well as his safety. One night after finally dozing off after getting Ed tucked in, I awoke to find him standing over me with an ominous look. My heart started pounding so fast I thought I would have a heart attack. I also had to hide all the kitchen knives when I discovered he had put two sharp knives in his robe pocket. This was as I was attempting to block the door to prevent him from wandering . . . he had knives in his pocket when he pushed me out of the way.

I know a lot of people think they can do it all, only time will tell if that remains true. Everyone must decide when or if they need to seek help. I got help first by having home aides come in, then adult day care, memory care and finally long-term care. I found that many, many times there will not be as much family support as you think. Somehow the siblings or grown children will not be able to help out for various reasons. However, these same family members will show up to criticize or second-guess every decision you've made. This is when you must stand firm. If necessary, you may have to limit contact and visitations with these family members. They do not know what you're going through. They haven't walked in your shoes. They haven't had sleepless nights or had to change adult diapers or change linen several times a day or lived in fear for their own safety.

In addition to being flexible, I found that a good sense of humor helps. Some of the things Ed said or did were just funny. When I laughed out loud, he would join in. We shared many happy moments filled with laughter. There were more of these moments once he was placed when I could just share time with him as his wife rather than being his full-time caregiver. It is also worth noting that you must take care of yourself, eat healthy, rest and keep up with your own doctor appointments. Try to find moments just for you. It is my wish for anyone going through this with a loved one that you find the best solution available to you, that you protect the dignity of your loved one and find those moments that bring you peace with the knowledge that you have done the best you could.

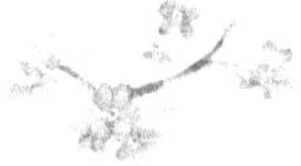

Appendix A

Tips for Engaging with Loved Ones with Dementia

1. Approach with calm body language and speak slowly and clearly.

2. Agree, do not argue.

3. Divert or distract. Do not attempt to reason. You cannot convince them they do not see or hear what they claim to see or hear.

4. Reminisce with them and try not ask, "Do you remember . . . ?"

5. Repeat things as many times as necessary. Do not say, "I told you already." Distract if necessary.

6. Don't ask open-ended questions. Give them simple choices like "tea or coffee?", or, ask questions that require a yes or no answer.

7. Create daily routines that they enjoy—puzzles, singing familiar songs, listening to music, looking at old photographs, coloring, etc.

8. Offer reassurance when needed—repeat calming words (e.g., "You're safe here").

9. Validate their feelings.

10. Encourage, do not condescend. Focus on what they can do, not what they can't.

Appendix B

Relaxation Ideas for Caregivers

- Listen to calming music or nature sounds
- Use aromatherapy (lavender, eucalyptus, chamomile)
- Relax with a weighted blanket
- Enjoy a warm bath with Epsom salts
- Read a book, poem, or short story
- Write in a journal for a few minutes
- Engage in a creative hobby (painting, knitting, gardening)
- Watch a feel-good movie or show
- Join a caregiver support group
- Talk with a friend or therapist
- Schedule regular "me time"
- Sip tea or coffee slowly, without multitasking

- Step outside for fresh air and sunlight
- Write down 3 things you're grateful for
- Do gentle yoga or stretching or deep breathing (4-7-8) exercises
- Take a walk in nature or a nearby park

Appendix C

Helpful Resources for Caregivers

Alzheimer's Association
www.alz.org
ph. 1-800-272-3900

Aging Care
www.agingcare.org
ph. 1-888-887-4593

Alzheimer's Foundation of America
www.Alzfdn.org
ph. 1-866-232-8484

Dementia Society
www.dementiasociety.org
ph. 1-800-DEMENTIA

National Institution on Aging
www.nia.nih.gov
ph. 1-800-222-2225

- Teepa Snow's Positive Approach to Care videos on YouTube
- *The 36-Hour Day* book by Nancy L. Mace, MA, and Peter V. Rabins, MD, MPH
- *Coach Broyles' Playbook for Alzheimer's Caregivers* by J. Frank Broyles.

Other helpful sources include:

- Local senior citizen centers
- Area Agencies on Aging
- Faith-based organizations
- Support groups at churches, hospitals, nursing homes
- Adult day care centers

About the Author

Judy Collier was born and raised in Philadelphia, PA. She was educated in the public school system and is a graduate of Temple University. Her employment throughout the years gave her the opportunity to live in several cities before returning to her hometown where she met and married Ed. She has one son and enjoys traveling as a retiree after many years of caregiving.

Acknowledgments

I am so thankful that God has placed me in a circle of supportive and caring people. I am grateful for my friend Michele Roberts who, unbeknownst to her, encouraged me to get up off my tail and do something productive. Since the passing of my husband I had gotten into a routine of just sitting around my house falling deeper into introvertism. She motivated me to get out, go to museums, the library, bookstores, etc. This prompted me to start typing out my journal. I appreciate our many long phone conversations and your hospitality whenever I visited.

I also thank my wonderful son, Marques Green, who took the time to read and critique my raw manuscript. With his eye for detail and inquisitive mind, he provided suggestions that immensely helped with clarity and the "pulling together" of the narrative. I love you unconditionally.

I am forever grateful to Beth Werner of Author Connections. It was her comments after reading my manuscript that motivated me to go public with this work when I considered just keeping it within my family. We met at just the right time in our lives, and I do believe it was not coincidental but was in divine order.

Finally, thanks to all the readers who may have found this little book helpful. I hope it guides you when you are looking for answers during your journey.

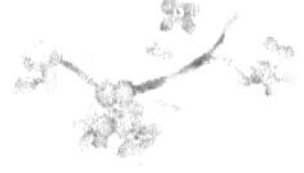